JULIE M. MONTGOMERY

Mindful Weight Loss

A Proven Guide to Rewire Your Brain to Reach Your Goals Faster

Contents

1

Introduction

There is a profound connection between the mind and the body. This transformative guide recognizes that weight management is not solely about diet and exercise but must be a holistic approach that engages the power of the mind. Thoughts, emotions, and habits intricately influence our relationship with food and our bodies. The power of mindfulness, meditation, positive thinking, and affirmations can be harnessed for lasting physical and mental well-being.

Mindfulness is a practice that involves being fully present and engaged in the current moment. By cultivating mindfulness, we gain an awareness of our emotions and thought patterns, laying the foundation for mindful eating and conscious decision-making. Meditation has neuroscientific underpinnings and understanding it can reshape our relationship with stress, cravings, and ultimately, our bodies. Positive thinking and affirmations illuminate the path to a healthier mindset, providing tools to silence the inner critic and reinforce positive beliefs to achieve lasting change.

This is an invitation to embrace empowerment, as you become equipped with valuable transformative tools. Your mind and thinking can become the driving force behind your weight loss success—a mindful and intentional way of living that nurtures mind and body simultaneously. Such a lifestyle shift fosters a sense of self-compassion, encouraging readers to approach their weight loss journey with patience, understanding, and an openness to the transformative power within.

2

Understanding the Mind-Body Connection

The mind and body, often treated as distinct entities, are woven together in a delicate dance that shapes our approach to weight management. It is within this nexus that mindfulness takes center stage, offering a holistic, empowering lens through which we can observe, understand, and ultimately reshape our behaviors.

Our thoughts, emotions, and mental habits play a pivotal role in shaping our behaviors, especially concerning food choices and eating patterns. Negative thought patterns, emotional triggers, and stress can lead to unhealthy eating habits, contributing to weight gain and hindering weight loss efforts. Mindfulness becomes a transformative tool, allowing us to observe our thoughts and emotions without judgment, fostering a heightened awareness of the factors influencing our eating behaviors. By understanding and reshaping thought patterns, we gain agency over our relationship with food.

In the pursuit of weight loss, understanding the intricate interplay between thoughts, emotions, and habits is paramount. Our relationship with food is profoundly influenced by the thoughts we harbor, the emotions we experience, and the habits we cultivate. Negative thought patterns, often rooted in self-criticism or a distorted body image, can lead to emotional distress and serve as triggers for unhealthy eating behaviors. Thoughts, as silent architects of our behaviors, shape the choices we make around food. Negative self-talk can create a cycle of emotional eating, where we turn to food for comfort or as a coping mechanism for stress, anxiety, or other emotional challenges. Conversely, positive thoughts can pave the way for mindful and intentional eating, fostering healthier habits.

Emotions act as potent catalysts in the realm of eating behaviors. Stress, a ubiquitous part of modern life, can trigger the release of cortisol, a hormone linked to increased appetite and cravings, particularly for comfort foods high in sugar and fat. Emotional states, whether joy, sadness, or boredom, often dictate food choices, influencing both the type and quantity of consumed foods.

Habits, deeply ingrained through repetition, further solidify the impact of thoughts and emotions on eating behaviors. Unconscious habits, such as reaching for snacks during television watching or engaging in mindless eating at social gatherings, can undermine weight loss efforts. Breaking these habits requires a conscious effort to rewire the thought patterns and emotional triggers that perpetuate them.

Mindfulness unravels the threads of thought, emotion, and habit. Meditation allows us to develop emotional regulation skills so we can navigate stressors more effectively, reducing the likelihood of stress-induced eating. Positive thinking emerges as a powerful force in reshaping thought patterns, fostering self-compassion, and promoting a healthier relationship with food. Affirmations will reinforce our positive thinking, ultimately rewiring our cognitive landscape to support sustained weight loss.

Mindful eating encourages a heightened awareness of our eating habits and the overall experience of consuming food. It means being fully present in the moment, cultivating a deep connection with the act of eating. This approach encourages us to engage all our senses—

savoring the flavors, textures, and aromas of each bite. Beyond mere physical nourishment, it encompasses the emotional and psychological aspects of the experience of eating.

By paying close attention to hunger and fullness cues, we develop a more intuitive relationship with our bodies, allowing them to distinguish between genuine hunger and emotional triggers. Mindful eating emphasizes the importance of slowing down during meals, savoring each bite, and fostering a non-judgmental awareness of one's thoughts and feelings related to food.

3

Science Supports Mindfulness and Weight Loss

At the intersection of brain function and behavior, research has unveiled compelling evidence supporting the efficacy of mindfulness practices in reshaping cognitive processes related to eating behaviors. Neural imaging studies showcase the tangible effects of mindfulness and meditation on brain regions associated with self-control, emotional regulation, and decision-making—crucial elements in the battle against overeating and unhealthy dietary patterns. These insights provide a scientific foundation for understanding how mindfulness influences our relationship with food and can empower us to make intentional, health-conscious choices.

At the heart of the neuroscientific understanding lies the concept of neuroplasticity, the brain's remarkable ability to adapt and reorganize itself in response to experiences and stimuli. Mindfulness and meditation are catalysts for this neural adaptation, influencing the structure and function of key brain regions associated with self-regulation, emotional processing, and decision-making.

Research has illuminated the role of the prefrontal cortex, the brain's executive center, in the practice of mindfulness. This region is crucial for impulse control, emotional regulation, and long-term planning—essential components in the realm of weight management. Mindfulness practices, such as focused attention on the breath or body sensations, have been shown to enhance prefrontal cortex activity, enhancing cognitive control, emotional regulation, and long-term planning. Studies demonstrate that mindfulness practices can lead to structural changes in the amygdala, resulting in reduced reactivity to emotional stimuli. This is particularly relevant in curbing emotional eating. Mindfulness and meditation also impact the insula, a brain region integral to interoception—the perception of internal bodily sensations. When we tune in to the physical sensations associated with cravings, such as the taste, texture, or smell of specific foods, we experience heightened awareness that allows us to respond to cravings with a more discerning, non-judgmental perspective, ultimately reducing the likelihood of succumbing to unhealthy temptations. Mindfulness practices deactivate the default mode network (DMN), a network associated with self-referential thinking and mind-wandering, thus diminishing ruminative thoughts about food. This shift in neural activity creates a mental space for deliberate, conscious decision-making around food. Additionally, studies reveal the modulation of the hippocampus, a region involved in memory and learning, by mindfulness practices. Enhanced hippocampal function may support the consolidation of positive habits and the formation of healthier routines related to diet and exercise.

Cravings, often a formidable hurdle in the weight loss journey, are intimately connected to the brain's reward circuitry. Mindfulness practices, such as focused attention on the breath or body sensations, bring about changes in the mesolimbic system—a key component of the reward pathway. Research indicates that mindfulness can modulate the release of dopamine, a neurotransmitter associated with pleasure and reward, thereby mitigating the intensity of cravings.

Neural imaging studies further illuminate the impact of mindfulness on the brain's response to food cues. By training the mind to respond more thoughtfully to stimuli, mindfulness diminishes the hyperactivity in the reward centers triggered by images of appetizing foods. This neural desensitization, coupled with heightened self-awareness, contributes to a more balanced and intentional approach to food consumption.

Meditation, similarly demonstrates neuroscientific benefits. Regular meditation has been linked to changes in gray matter density, particularly in brain regions associated with self-awareness, compassion, and emotional regulation. These structural alterations contribute to the cultivation of a mindful mindset that is pivotal in navigating the challenges of weight management.

In essence, the integration of mindfulness practices into the weight loss journey encapsulates a profound recalibration of the brain's responses to cravings and decision making processes. Mindfulness acts as a cognitive ally, rewiring the brain's landscape to neurologically empower us with the tools of intention, resilience, and a renewed sense of control.

4

Cultivating Mindful Eating Habits

M indful eating is not a diet but a conscious and intentional approach to nourishing our bodies. It is a transformative shift—one that transcends calorie counting and embraces a holistic approach to well-being. Each bite is an opportunity to savor life and nourish not just the body but the soul. The following is a guide to get you started

Eliminate Distractions

Create a mindful eating environment by turning off screens, putting away electronic devices, and sitting down at a designated eating space. Minimizing distractions allows you to fully engage with your meal.

Portion Awareness

Pay attention to portion sizes. Use smaller plates and bowls to encourage mindful portions. This helps in preventing overeating and promotes awareness of satiety.

Eat Without Judgment

Release judgment intentionally about good or bad foods. Approach eating with self-compassion and without guilt. Acknowledge that all foods can be a part of a balanced and mindful diet.

Begin with Presence

Start your meal with a moment of presence. Take a few deep breaths, appreciate the appearance and aroma of your food.

Mindful Bites

Chew slowly and savor each bite. Focus on the textures and flavors. This not only enhances the eating experience but also allows your brain to register fullness more effectively.

Engage Your Senses

Utilize your senses to connect with your food. Notice the colors, smells, and textures. Engaging multiple senses enhances the sensory experience of eating.

Pause Between Bites

Put your utensils down between bites. This simple act introduces a natural pause, allowing you to check in with your body's signals of hunger and fullness.

Listen to Your Body

Tune into your body's cues. Eat when you're hungry, and stop when you're satisfied. Recognize the difference between physical hunger and emotional cravings.

Express Gratitude

Take a moment after your meal to express gratitude for the nour-ishment you've received. This can be a mindful way to conclude your eating experience positively.

Reflect on Choices

After your meal, reflect on the choices you made and how your body feels. This reflection fosters self-awareness and helps you make mindful choices in future meals.

Incorporating these practical tips into your eating routines can foster a more mindful approach to food, promoting not only physical well-being but also a deeper connection with the act of nourishing your body.

Along with these guidelines, you can add mindful eating exercises to help train your brain in this new appreciation of food.

The Raisin Exercise

A single raisin can cultivate deep awareness of the eating experience. Take a moment to examine the raisin—its texture, color, and shape. Hold it in your hand, feeling its weight and contours. Bring it to your nose, inhaling deeply to capture its scent. As you place the raisin in your mouth, savor the taste and notice the sensations as you chew slowly. (Alternatives: use an almond or olive)

Five Senses Check-In

Begin your meal with a brief check-in of each of your five senses. Take a moment to observe the visual aspects of your food—the colors, shapes, and arrangement. Inhale deeply to appreciate the aroma. Run your fingertips around the edges of your plate, feel the weight and smoothness of your fork, the texture of your napkin. Listen to the sounds of your eating experience, whether it's the crunch of vegetables or the softness of bread. Finally, savor the flavors with each bite.

Mindful Breathing Between Bites

After taking a bite or two, put down your utensil and take a slow, deep breath. Use this moment to observe any sensations in your body and check in with your level of fullness. This practice allows your brain to catch up with your body's signals of satiety and encourages a conscious pace of eating, preventing mindless over-consumption.

5

The Power of Meditation for Weight Loss

Meditation serves as a powerful tool for stress reduction by offering a structured and intentional approach to quieting the mind and fostering a sense of inner calm. In the midst of our fast-paced and often chaotic lives, stress can accumulate, leading to physical and mental tension. Meditation provides a dedicated space to redirect attention inward, allowing us to observe our thoughts without judgment.

Moreover, meditation triggers the relaxation response, activating the parasympathetic nervous system. This physiological shift leads to decreased heart rate, lowered blood pressure, and reduced levels of stress hormones. The rhythmic and intentional nature of meditation induces a state of deep relaxation, counteracting the physiological arousal associated with stress.

Through techniques such as focused breathing, guided imagery, or mindfulness meditation, we learn to anchor our awareness in the present moment. This deliberate focus helps cultivate an increased capacity to detach from stressors, viewing them with a more objective and less emotionally charged perspective. Over time, this heightened resilience fosters not only stress reduction but also a holistic sense of well-being.

Stress, Cortisol, and Weight gain

The intricate link between stress, cortisol, and weight gain is a well-established facet of the complex interplay between the mind and body. Stress, whether acute or chronic, triggers a cascade of physiological responses, with cortisol, often referred to as the stress hormone, playing a central role in this intricate connection.

When the body perceives a stressor, the hypothalamus signals the release of corticotropin-releasing hormone (CRH). This, in turn, prompts the pituitary gland to release adrenocorticotropic hormone (ACTH), which signals the adrenal glands to produce cortisol. Cortisol is a potent regulator of metabolism, immune function, and the body's response to stress. In the short term, this stress response is adaptive, preparing the body to face a perceived threat. However, chronic stress can lead to sustained elevation of cortisol levels, and prolonged exposure to elevated cortisol has several implications for weight management.

Appetite and Cravings

Cortisol influences appetite regulation by interacting with the brain's reward centers. It can lead to increased cravings, particularly for high-calorie and comfort foods. This response is part of the body's evolutionary mechanism to replenish energy stores in the face of a perceived threat.

Abdominal Fat Accumulation

Cortisol promotes the storage of fat, particularly visceral fat, which accumulates around abdominal organs. This distribution is associated with an increased risk of metabolic conditions such as insulin resistance and cardiovascular disease.

Blood Sugar Regulation

Cortisol plays a role in maintaining blood sugar levels by promoting gluconeogenesis, the production of glucose from non-carbohydrate sources. Elevated cortisol can lead to increased blood sugar levels, contributing to insulin resistance and the potential for fat storage.

Metabolic Rate and Muscle Mass

Chronic stress and elevated cortisol levels can negatively impact metabolic rate and muscle mass. Cortisol may interfere with the body's ability to build and maintain lean muscle, which is metabolically active and contributes to overall energy expenditure.

Insulin Sensitivity

Cortisol can reduce insulin sensitivity, impairing the body's ability to regulate blood sugar effectively. Insulin resistance is a key factor in the development of obesity and metabolic syndrome.

The good news is that mindfulness practices have been shown to help regulate cortisol levels. The parasympathetic nervous system is no longer in fight, flight, or freeze mode as breathing and other exercises provide calm redirection. As a result, mindfulness can be employed as a powerful regulator in times of stress.

Guided Meditation Exercises

Here are five guided meditation exercises that will let your body know you don't have to fight the bear or run from the bear. Experience the calm tranquility you need to convince your cortisol you are safe.

Body Scan Meditation

Find a quiet and comfortable space to sit or lie down. Close your eyes and bring your attention to your breath.

Begin to scan your body from head to toe, paying attention to each part. Notice any areas of tension or discomfort, and with each exhale, release the tension.

Progressively move through your body, bringing awareness to each region. This exercise promotes relaxation by grounding you in the present moment and releasing physical tension.

Loving-Kindness Meditation

Sit comfortably and close your eyes. Start by directing feelings of love and kindness toward yourself. Repeat phrases like "May I be happy, may I be healthy, may I be safe, may I be at ease."

Extend these wishes to others, beginning with someone close to you, then gradually expanding to acquaintances, difficult individuals, and eventually to all beings.

This meditation cultivates feelings of compassion and connection, fostering a sense of inner peace and relaxation.

Visualization Meditation

Close your eyes and imagine a peaceful scene, such as a beach, forest, or meadow. Spend time picturing the details—the colors, sounds, and smells.

As you visualize, engage your senses. Feel the warmth of the sun, hear the rustle of leaves, and inhale the fresh air.

Use visualization meditation to transport your mind to your serene place any time you need relaxation or a mental escape from stressors.

Breathing Exercises

Focus on your breath, inhaling deeply through your nose and exhaling through your mouth. Lengthen your breath, making each inhalation and exhalation smooth and controlled.

Try different breath patterns, such as diaphragmatic breathing or the 4-7-8 technique (inhale for a count of 4, hold for 7, exhale for 8).

Deep breathing exercises activate the body's relaxation response, calming the nervous system and promoting a sense of tranquility. They communicate safety and security to your brain and body. *"You don't have to fight the bear. You don't have to run from the bear. There is no bear."*

Mindfulness Meditation

Sit in a comfortable position and bring your attention to your breath. Observe the natural flow of your breath without attempting to change it.

As thoughts arise, acknowledge them without judgment and gently return your focus to your breath.

Mindfulness meditation encourages non-judgmental awareness, helping you become present in the moment and reducing stress by disengaging from distracting thoughts.

Experiment with these exercises to discover which resonates most with you, and consider integrating them into your routine for a more peaceful state of being.

6

Rewiring Thought Patterns

Negative thought patterns can significantly impede weight loss efforts by influencing behaviors, emotions, and our overall mindset. These patterns often manifest as self-critical thoughts, doubts, or pessimism regarding one's ability to achieve weight loss goals.

When we harbor negative beliefs about our bodies or abilities, we may turn to food as a coping mechanism for stress, anxiety, or low self-esteem. Emotional eating can lead to the consumption of calorie-dense and nutrient-poor foods.

Moreover, negative thought patterns can erode motivation and self-discipline. Believing that weight loss is impossible or that past failures define future outcomes can create a self-fulfilling prophecy. We become demotivated, making it challenging to adhere to healthy habits such as regular exercise or mindful eating.

Negative thoughts also impact stress levels, contributing to the release of cortisol. Chronic stress, fueled by negative thought patterns, creates a cycle where stress triggers unhealthy eating habits, leading to weight gain, leading to more negative thoughts, more stress and so on.

The impact of negative thought patterns extends to the physiological level as well. Studies suggest that chronic stress and negative emotions can disrupt hormonal balance, influencing appetite regulation and metabolism.

Addressing negative thought patterns is crucial for sustainable weight loss. Cognitive-behavioral strategies, mindfulness practices, and positive affirmations help reframe negative thoughts, build self-efficacy, and cultivate a healthier relationship with food and our bodies. We are then better equipped to make nourishing choices and navigate challenges with resilience.

Techniques for Fostering a Positive Mindset and Self-Image

Several techniques can be employed to cultivate positivity and build a more constructive view of oneself.

Positive Affirmations

Regularly engage in positive self-talk by incorporating affirmations into your daily routine. Affirmations are positive statements that reflect your goals, strengths, and self-worth. Repeatedly affirming these positive beliefs can gradually rewire your thinking to reinforce an optimistic self-image.

Gratitude Practice

Cultivate a habit of gratitude by reflecting on the positive aspects of your life. Regularly jot down or mentally acknowledge things you are thankful for. This practice shifts your focus from what may be lacking to what is abundant in your life.

Visualization

Use visualization techniques to picture your goals and envision positive outcomes. Imagine yourself succeeding, achieving your aspirations, and embodying the qualities you admire. Visualization enhances self-belief and creates a mental blueprint for positive experiences.

Mindfulness Meditation

Practice mindfulness meditation to stay present and non-judgmentally aware of your thoughts and feelings. Mindfulness helps detach from negative thought patterns, allowing you to observe them without getting entangled. Over time, this builds more accepting and positive neural pathways.

Challenge Negative Thoughts

Actively challenge and reframe negative thoughts. When negative self-talk arises, question its validity and replace it with more balanced and constructive thoughts. This cognitive restructuring helps break the cycle of pessimism and builds a more positive internal dialogue.

Self-Compassion

Develop self-compassion by treating yourself with the same kindness and understanding that you would offer to a friend. Embrace imperfections as part of the human experience, and recognize that setbacks do not define your worth.

Surround Yourself with Positivity

Foster positive relationships and surround yourself with people who uplift and support you. Engage in activities that bring joy and fulfillment. A positive external environment reinforces a constructive internal mindset.

Set Realistic Goals

Establish realistic and achievable goals. Break larger objectives into smaller, manageable steps, celebrating each accomplishment along the way. Attaining realistic goals boosts confidence and contributes to a positive self-image.

Practice Self-Care

Prioritize self-care activities that nourish your physical, emotional, and mental well-being. Taking care of yourself well signals self-worth and contributes to a positive self-image.

Seek Professional Support

If negative thought patterns persist and significantly impact your well-being, consider seeking support from a therapist or counselor. Professional guidance can provide personalized strategies to address underlying issues and promote a more positive mindset.

By incorporating these techniques into your daily life, you can gradually build a positive mindset, fostering positivity, self-compassion, and a healthier self-image. Remember that while building a positive mindset is a continuous process that requires practice and self-reflection, the result is new neural pathways in your brain that support and empower you.

Incorporating Positive Affirmations into Daily Routines

Incorporating positive affirmations into daily routines is a powerful practice for cultivating a positive mindset and enhancing overall well-being. Here are several ways to seamlessly integrate affirmations into your everyday life.

Morning Rituals

Begin your day with positive affirmations. Whether spoken aloud or silently in your mind, affirmations can set a positive tone for the day. Repeat statements that resonate with your goals, self-worth, and intentions for the day ahead.

Mirror Affirmations

Stand in front of a mirror and recite affirmations while looking at yourself. This technique enhances the connection between the affirmation and your self-perception. Speak affirmations about your strengths, capabilities, and the positive qualities you embody.

Affirmation Cards or Sticky Notes

Create a set of affirmation cards or write affirmations on sticky notes. Place them in prominent locations where you'll see them frequently—on your bathroom mirror, computer monitor, or refrigerator. These visual cues will serve as reminders throughout the day.

Incorporate Affirmations into Mindfulness Practices

Integrate affirmations into mindfulness or meditation sessions. Repeat affirmations during moments of stillness and reflection. This can enhance the impact of the affirmation by aligning it with a focused and calm state of mind.

Use Affirmation Apps

Leverage technology by using affirmation apps that send reminders or notifications throughout the day. Set a schedule for affirmations to pop up on your phone, providing a digital prompt for positive thinking.

Create an Affirmation Journal

Dedicate a section of your journal to positive affirmations. Write down affirmations that resonate with you. There is something incredibly powerful in writing down our thoughts on paper with our own hand. They become more real somehow and we embrace them more strongly.

Revisit your affirmations regularly, reflect on your progress, and update them as your journey evolves.

Incorporate Affirmations into Daily Tasks

Connect affirmations with routine activities. Repeat them while commuting, exercising, or doing household chores. Associating affirmations with daily tasks helps integrate positive thinking seamlessly into your routine.

Affirmation Breaks

Take short breaks throughout the day to pause and recite affirmations. This can be particularly beneficial during moments of stress or when facing challenges, providing a mental reset and reinforcing positive thinking.

Affirmations Before Sleep

End your day on a positive note by reciting affirmations before bedtime. This can create a positive mindset as you transition into sleep, influencing your subconscious mind during the night.

Affirmation Group or Partner

Share affirmations with a friend or family member. This sense of community can enhance the impact of affirmations and provide mutual support.

Remember that consistency is key when incorporating affirmations into daily routines. Choose affirmations that resonate with you personally and adapt them as needed to align with your evolving goals and mindset. Over time, this practice can contribute to a more positive and empowering outlook on life.

7

Affirmations for Weight Loss Success

Personalized affirmations for weight loss goals should be positive and empowering, and tailored to address specific challenges and aspirations. These affirmations serve to reinforce a positive mindset, boost motivation, and support behavioral changes. Here are a few to get you started.

Positive Body Image

"I love and appreciate my body at every stage of my weight loss journey."

"My body is strong, and I am grateful for its resilience and capabilities."

Empowerment in Choices

"I make mindful choices that nourish and support my health and well-being."

"Every healthy choice I make brings me closer to my weight loss goals."

Persistence and Resilience

"I am resilient, and I persist in the face of challenges."

"Obstacles are opportunities for growth, and I overcome them with determination."

Affirming Progress

"I celebrate every small achievement on my weight loss journey."

"Each day, I am moving closer to my ideal weight and a healthier me."

Overcoming Emotional Eating

"I am in control of my emotions, and I choose nourishing alternatives to cope with stress."

"Food does not define my emotions; I find healthy ways to manage stress and anxiety."

Enjoying the Process

"I find joy in the journey of transforming my body and mind."

"Each step I take toward weight loss is a step toward a happier and healthier life."

Boosting Self-Confidence

"I am confident in my ability to achieve my weight loss goals."

"My self-worth is not determined by my weight; I am valuable and deserving of health."

Affirming Physical Activity

"Exercise is a gift to my body, and I enjoy the benefits of movement."

"I prioritize physical activity, and it contributes to my overall well-being."

Mindful Eating

"I savor each bite, eating with mindfulness and gratitude."

"My body knows when it's satisfied, and I listen to its signals."

Future Vision

"I visualize myself at my ideal weight, living a vibrant and healthy life."

"My future is filled with energy, confidence, and a strong, healthy body."

These personalized affirmations can be adapted to resonate with your experiences and challenges. Regular repetition of these affirmations, combined with other healthy lifestyle practices, contribute to a positive mindset and successful weight loss outcomes.

Incorporating Affirmations into Meditation and Mindfulness Practices

Incorporating affirmations into meditation and mindfulness practices can enhance the effectiveness of both techniques, fostering a positive and focused state of mind. Here's a guide on how to seamlessly integrate affirmations into your meditation and mindfulness routine.

Set an Intention

Begin your meditation or mindfulness session by setting a clear intention. Identify the specific aspect of your life, mindset, or well-being that you want to focus on. This intention will guide the choice of affirmations.

Find a Comfortable Position

Choose a comfortable and quiet space for your practice. Sit or lie down in a relaxed position, allowing your body to be at ease.

Start with Mindful Breathing

Begin your session with a few minutes of mindful breathing to center your attention. Focus on the sensation of your breath—inhaling and exhaling—allowing yourself to be fully present in the moment.

Introduce Affirmations Gradually

Once you've established a sense of calm, introduce affirmations gradually. Start with a positive and concise affirmation related to your intention. For example, if your intention is self-love, an affirmation could be, "I am deserving of love and kindness."

Repeat Affirmations Mindfully

As you incorporate affirmations, repeat them mindfully. Align the words of the affirmation with your breath, saying the affirmation during the inhalation and exhalation. This rhythmic repetition enhances the integration of affirmations into your meditative state.

Visualize Affirmations

Combine affirmations with visualization. As you repeat the affirmation, create a mental image that corresponds to the words. For instance, if your affirmation is about achieving a goal, visualize yourself successfully reaching that goal.

Feel the Affirmation

Engage your senses by evoking the feeling associated with the affirmation. Allow the positive emotion or energy of the affirmation to permeate your body and mind. This sensory connection enhances the impact of the affirmation.

Maintain Focus

Keep your attention on the present moment and the affirmations. If your mind starts to wander, gently guide your focus back to the words and sensations associated with the affirmations.

Conclude with Silence

Towards the end of your session, let go of the repetition and sit in silent mindfulness. Allow the positive energy cultivated by the affirmations to linger as you embrace a few moments of stillness.

Reflect on the Experience

After your meditation or mindfulness practice, take a moment to reflect on the experience. Notice any shifts in your mindset or emotional state. Reflecting on the impact of affirmations reinforces their positive influence.

Consistency is key when incorporating affirmations into meditation and mindfulness practices. Regular repetition of affirmations in a mindful context gradually reshapes thought patterns and contributes to a positive and empowered mindset over time.

Tracking Progress and Adjusting Affirmations

Tracking progress and adjusting affirmations is a dynamic process that involves self-reflection and adaptation. Here's a guide on how to effectively track progress and modify affirmations as needed.

Set Clear Objectives

Clearly define your goals and intentions related to the affirmations. Whether it's improving self-esteem, managing stress, or achieving specific milestones, having well-defined objectives provides a basis for tracking progress.

Journaling

Maintain a journal where you record your affirmations, along with your thoughts and feelings associated with them. This written documentation provides a tangible record of your journey, allowing you to track changes over time.

Monitor Emotional Responses

Pay attention to your emotional responses when repeating affirmations. Note any shifts in mood, changes in self-perception, or improvements in overall well-being. Positive emotional responses indicate progress.

Evaluate Behavioral Changes

Assess any behavioral changes that align with your affirmations. If, for example, your affirmation focuses on healthy habits, observe whether you are making positive choices in your daily life that reflect this intention.

Seek Feedback from Others

Engage in open conversations with trusted friends, family members, or mentors about your progress. External perspectives provide valuable insights and offer a different lens through which to evaluate your journey.

Identify Areas of Growth

Recognize areas where you have experienced growth or positive changes. Celebrate achievements, no matter how small, and acknowledge the effort you've put into fostering a positive mindset.

Detect Areas for Adjustment

Be attentive to areas where affirmations may need adjustment. If certain affirmations no longer resonate or if new challenges arise, consider modifying the language or focus to better address your evolving needs.

Modify Affirmations Gradually

When adjustments are needed, modify affirmations gradually. Introduce changes one at a time to allow for a smooth transition. Focus on creating affirmations that align more closely with your current mindset and goals.

Maintain a Growth Mindset

Embrace a growth mindset that views challenges as opportunities for learning and adaptation. If certain affirmations are not yielding the desired results, view it as an opportunity to refine and improve your approach.

Periodic Review and Revision

Schedule periodic reviews of your affirmations and overall progress—weekly or monthly. This routine creates a structured opportunity to gauge the effectiveness of your affirmations.

Stay Open to Exploration

Be open to exploring new affirmations or adjusting the focus of existing ones. As you evolve, your affirmations may naturally shift to align with your changing priorities and aspirations.

Remember that personal growth is a dynamic and ongoing process. By consistently tracking progress, staying attuned to your needs, and adjusting affirmations as necessary, you can cultivate a positive and adaptive mindset that supports your overall well-being.

8

Building Sustainable Habits

Building sustainable habits is crucial for long-term success and well-being, as it establishes a foundation of positive routines that contribute to lasting personal growth and fulfillment.

Consistency in Behavior

Habits provide a framework for consistent behavior which helps to regulate calorie intake, maintain physical activity levels, and sustain the overall balance necessary for effective weight management. Positive habits reduce the likelihood of erratic and impulsive choices that can hinder progress.

Automatic Decision-Making

When healthy habits become ingrained, we are more likely to make nutritious food choices, engage in physical activity, and prioritize self-care without relying on sheer willpower. This automaticity streamlines efforts, reducing cognitive load and making it more feasible to maintain a healthy lifestyle over the long term.

Behavioral Reinforcement

Habits act as a form of behavioral reinforcement, shaping attitudes and preferences toward healthier options. Over time, this positive reinforcement contributes to a sustainable mindset, wherein we derive intrinsic satisfaction from making healthy choices, reinforcing a positive feedback loop crucial for maintaining long-term weight management success. Conversely, breaking negative habits and replacing them with healthier alternatives disrupts detrimental patterns and contributes to a more positive lifestyle.

Mindful Habit-Building Strategies for Exercise

Mindful habit-building strategies for exercise would include beginning with a manageable exercise routine to avoid overwhelm and setting realistic and achievable goals. Break larger objectives into smaller milestones, celebrating each accomplishment and maintaining motivation for continued progress.

Understanding your personal motivation will fuel lasting commitment so identify and connect with your intrinsic reasons for exercise. Engage in mindful movement by paying attention to the sensations, breath, and muscle engagement during exercise. This fosters a deeper connection with your body and enhances the overall experience.

Mindful Habit-Building Strategies for Nutrition

Mindful habit-building strategies for nutrition include tuning into your body's cues, eating when hungry and stopping when satisfied. Plan and prepare meals in advance to avoid impulsive and less nutritious choices. Drinking water mindfully throughout the day to stay hydration supports overall well-being and can contribute to a more balanced approach to food.

Mindful Habit-Building Strategies for Self-Care

Mindful habit-building strategies for self-care include prioritizing sufficient, restful sleep with a consistent bedtime routine. Setting boundaries protects your time and energy. Saying no when needed and prioritizing self-care activities contribute to a healthier work-life balance. Dedicate time to hobbies and activities you enjoy. Pleasurable pursuits contribute to overall life satisfaction and support emotional well-being.

Developing a Mindful Approach to Setbacks and Challenges

Cultivate Self-Awareness

Reflect on your thoughts, emotions, and reactions to recognize patterns of thinking and behavior.

Stay Present in the Moment

Train yourself to stay present during challenges. When faced with setbacks, consciously bring your focus to the current moment. Avoid getting lost in past regrets or future anxieties, allowing for a more constructive response.

Cultivate a Non-Judgmental Mindset

Release the habit of labeling situations as good or bad. Adopt a non-judgmental mindset to view setbacks as opportunities for growth. This shift in perspective allows for more objective problem-solving and reduces emotional reactivity.

Practice Mindful Breathing

Use mindful breathing as a tool to stay calm during challenges. Focus on your breath, inhaling and exhaling slowly. This practice regulates the nervous system, (reminds it that you don't need to fight the bear or run away from the bear) promoting a more composed and thoughtful response.

Develop Self-Compassion

Be kind to yourself in the face of setbacks. Cultivate self-compassion by treating yourself with the same understanding and support you would offer to a friend. Acknowledge that everyone encounters challenges and mistakes are part of the learning process.

Learn from Setbacks

Approach setbacks as opportunities for learning. Reflect on the lessons each challenge presents. What insights can you gain from the experience, and how can you apply them to future situations?

9

Nurturing a Mindful Lifestyle

Nurturing a mindful lifestyle involves cultivating intentional awareness in daily activities, fostering a deeper connection between mind and body, and making conscious choices that prioritize overall well-being. Integrating mindfulness, meditation, positive thinking, and affirmations helps us develop a holistic and empowered approach to weight management by harnessing the power of the mind-body connection.

Step-by-Step Guide to Creating a Personalized Mindfulness Plan for Sustained Success in Weight Management

1. Define your goals and intentions for weight management. Be specific about what you want to achieve and how mindfulness will support your journey.
2. Reflect on your current lifestyle, habits, and stressors. Identify areas where mindfulness can be incorporated, considering both eating behaviors and physical activity.
3. Select mindfulness practices that resonate with you. This may include meditation, mindful eating, or deep-breathing exercises.

Tailor your choices to align with your preferences and lifestyle.

4. Integrate mindfulness into your daily routine. Set aside dedicated time for practice, whether it's a morning meditation, mindful mealtime, or evening reflection. Consistency is key for long-term success.

5. Employ mindful eating habits. Pay attention to the sensory experience of eating.

6. Develop positive affirmations that align with your weight loss goals. Use empowering statements to reinforce a healthy mindset and counteract negative self-talk.

7. Incorporate visualization into your routine. Picture yourself achieving your weight management goals, envision the positive impact on your health, and visualize the steps you'll take to get there.

8. Choose exercises that allow for mindful movement and pay attention to the sensations in your body, your breath, and the present moment during physical activity.

9. Explore mindfulness apps or resources that align with your preferences. Whether guided meditations, affirmations, or mindfulness exercises, leverage technology to support your mindfulness journey.

10. Keep a mindfulness journal to track your progress, thoughts, and feelings. Reflect on challenges, successes, and insights gained through your mindfulness practices.

11. Schedule regular self-check-ins to assess your mindfulness practices and their impact on your weight management journey. Adjust your plan as needed, acknowledging what works well and areas for improvement.

12. Anticipate challenges and setbacks. Develop strategies to navigate them mindfully, whether it's stress, emotional eating triggers, or disruptions to your routine. Learn from setbacks and adjust your

approach.

13. Celebrate milestones and achievements along the way. Acknowledge your progress, no matter how small, and use positive reinforcement to stay motivated.

14. Engage with a supportive community, whether online or in-person. Share your mindfulness journey, exchange insights, and seek guidance when needed.

15. Evolve Your Plan: As your weight management journey progresses, evolve your mindfulness plan. Adjust practices, set new goals, and continue refining your approach to ensure sustained success.

By following this step-by-step guide, you can create a personalized mindfulness plan that aligns with your unique preferences and supports your sustained success in weight management. Remember, mindfulness is a lifelong journey, and adapting your plan over time is integral to lasting positive change.

And as you continue to learn and practice mindfulness, neuroplasticity is at work supporting your efforts. Your brain is literally being rewired to encourage you and empower you to the life you desire.

Resources

Asadollahi, T., Khakpour, S., Ahmadi, F., Seyedeh, L.,Tahami, Matoo, S., Bermas, H.
   (2015). Effectiveness of mindfulness training and dietary regime on weight loss in
   obese people. Journal of Medicine and Life, v.8(Spec Iss 4). Retrieved from PubMed
   Database.

Chumachenko, S., Cali, R. J., Rosal, M. C., Allison, J. J., Person, S., Ziedonis, D. M.,
   Nephew, B. C., Moore, C. M., Zhang, N., King, J. A., & Fulwiler, C. E. (2021). Keeping
   weight off: Mindfulness-Based Stress Reduction alters amygdala functional
   connectivity during weight loss maintenance in a randomized control trial. PLOS
   ONE, 16(1), e0244847. https://doi.org/10.1371/journal.pone.0244847

Dunn, C., Haubenreiser, M., Johnson, M., Nordby, K., Aggarwal, S., Myer, S., & Thomas,
   C. (2018). Mindfulness approaches and weight loss, weight mainte-nance, and weight
   regain. Current Obesity Reports, 7(1), 37–49. https://doi.org/10.100

7/s13679-018-
  0299-6

Marchand, William R. (2014 Jul 28). Neural mechanisms of mindfulness and meditation:
  Evidence from neuroimaging studies. World of Radiology, 6(7): 471–479. Retrieved
    from PubMed Database.

O'Reilly, Gillian A., Cook, Lauren., Sprujit-Metz, Donna., and Black, David S. (2014 Mar
    18). Mindfulness-Based Interventions for Obesity-Related Eating Behaviors: A
    Literature Review. Obes Rev. 10.1111/obr.12156.

Seaver, M. (2023, August 9). What mindfulness does to your brain: The Science of
    Neuroplasticity. Real Simple. https://www.realsimple.com/health/mind
    mood/mindfulness-improves-brain-health-neuroplasticity

Warren, J., Smith, N., & Ashwell, M. (2017). A structured literature review on the role of
  mindfulness, mindful eating and intuitive eating in changing eating behaviours:
  effectiveness and associated potential mechanisms. Nutrition Research Reviews,
    30(2), 272–283. https://doi.org/10.1017/s0954422417000154